I0436778

Fitness Attack
101 Tips, Tricks, Do's, Don'ts and Other Random Thoughts from the Master of Fitness.

by Amy McIntyre

Written by Amy McIntyre
Edited by Joan Lekens & Scott Sigler
Designed by Chris McIntyre
Cover Design by Chris McIntyre
Photography by Michael Gomez

Copyright © 2007 by Amy McIntyre and WithAmyMac.com

All rights reserved. No part of this book may be reproduced without written permission from the publisher, except by a reviewer who may quote brief passages or reproduce illustrations in a review with appropriate credits; nor may any part of this book be reproduced, stored in a retrieval system, or transmitted in any form or by any means -- electronic, mechanical, photocopying, recording, or other -- without written permission from the publisher.

The information in this book is true and complete to the best of our knowledge. All recommendations are made without guarantee on the part of the author or publisher. The author and publisher disclaim any liability in connection with the use of this information. For additional information please contact Amy McIntyre at amy@withamymac.com

Books are available for special, premium and promotional uses and for customized editions. For further information, please email Amy McIntyre.

ISBN: 978-1-4357-0456-5

Acknowledgements

To my husband, who encouraged me to become Amy Mac and all that would come with it. Without your support, love and technical knowledge, none of this would be possible.

Special thanks to Scott Sigler and Joan Lekens for providing invaluable input on my first publication.

To my parents, family, friends, clients and audience... I am so grateful for all of your support (love, hugs and listens). I only hope that I have given you half as much as you have given me.

FITNESS ATTACK

Table of Contents

Introduction

Consult Your Physician

Tips 1-25

Tips 26-50

Tips 51-75

Tips 76-101

Introduction

In 2005, I became a personal trainer after years of dancing, rowing and enjoying time in the gym. I wanted to have a hand in helping individuals fight obesity and share my enthusiasm for health and fitness. In June 2006, I started Fitness Attack with Amy Mac, a 60 second health and fitness audio podcast. It became popular and successful much faster than I had imagined (thanks to my husband and PodShow). I am so excited to share my knowledge and passion with my clients and audience. This book is made possible by all of those who have listened, watched, supported, trusted and now read what I have to say about health and fitness.

Consult Your Physician

All information contained within this book and its accompanying shows and website, withamymac.com, is for informational purposes only. It is not intended to diagnose, treat, cure or prevent any health problem - nor is it intended to replace the advice of any health care professional. Please be advised that you are solely responsible for the way this information is perceived and utilized. We do not assume any liability for any injuries or health problems that might occur due to the use of these properties or the advice contained in them. Please see your physician before changing your diet or starting an exercise program. Discontinue any exercise that causes you pain or severe discomfort and consult a medical expert.

Tips 1-25

Fitness Attack

Water

Drinking water is incredibly important! If you are interested in losing weight, water is even more important. The average person needs to consume 96 oz. per day. The number increases if you are trying to lose weight or are working out. You should drink an additional 8 oz. per 25 lbs. you want to lose. Don't forget- anything you sweat out has to be replaced! The best way to consume water is to carry around a water bottle all day. You'll be amazed how natural it is to drink that much! Don't like the taste of water? You can always add those sugar-free flavor packs to add a little punch.

Amy Mac's Hints...

Tips to Drinking Enough Water:
- Carry a Water Bottle All Day
- Drink a Full Glass Before Each Meal
- Substitute Carbonated Beverages for Water

Where to find more Information:

- *The Benefits of Water - www.clevelandclinic.org*
- *Thirst Can Signal Dehydration - www.wistv.com*

Multivitamins

It is one of the most debated topics in health and fitness. Do vitamins really make a difference? There is a great deal of research that shows taking a daily multi-vitamin is a great supplement for some vitamins and minerals that may be lacking in your diet. It will help keep your body from having a vitamin deficiency and help promote overall health. Your diet plays a huge role in this, as well. If you are a healthy, well-rounded eater a simple daily vitamin is all you need. If you are a vegetarian, have a high protein diet or have specific dietary restrictions, you may need much more of some and much less of others. That's when a doctor or dietitian can assess your needs and give you specific recommendations. There is such a thing as overdoing vitamins, so self-diagnosing and self-prescribing can become a problem. If you're careful and consistent, a multivitamin can be beneficial to your overall health. Be smart; do your own research so you can honestly understand why you are taking what you're taking. Also remember to keep your age, diet, workout routine and health goals in mind.

Where to find more Information:
- *Vitamins - www.harvard.edu*
- *The Benefits of Dietary Supplements - www.crnusa.org*

Walking

Looking to burn a few more calories? Walking may be your answer. The average person walks around three miles a day. If you're looking to lose a few pounds, up that to five miles a day which is roughly 10,000 steps. Walking is an easy form of exercise that's easily forgotten in this convenience-driven world. The pedometer is a great way to keep track of your progress. Studies have shown that by just wearing a pedometer, you will walk more. Go ahead - take a few more steps today than you did yesterday. So many opportunities to squeeze in a few more steps!

Amy Mac's Hints...

Tips to Taking More Steps:

- Take the stairs, not the elevator.
- Park in the back of the parking lot.
- Walk around the block while you talk on your cell phone!
- Don't forget to walk to the market or walk the dog

Where to find more Information:

- *The Walking Site - www.thewalkingsite.com*
- *Walking for Health - www.ramblers.org.uk*
- *Walking - www.aarp.org*

Blueberries

For those of you who haven't heard, blueberries have some fantastic qualities! Blueberries are the fruit with the highest antioxidants. This means that they are constantly working to rid your body of free radicals that can cause numerous health problems. Blueberries have been found to fight cancer, be low in fat and calories, and they taste great. They are also high in Vitamin C and fiber. In laboratory studies, they were found to help in the anti-aging process and may help to reduce the buildup of the bad cholesterol "LDL." They're good for your skin, your health and maybe even your mental health. Now, no ONE thing is a cure all, but it sounds like adding blueberries to your diet is a great idea. One cup per day was the average amount used most in the studies and that equals only 81 calories!

Amy Mac's Hints...

Simple Blueberry Recipe Ideas:

- Add blueberries to plain, vanilla or strawberry yogurt
- Add blueberries to vanilla pudding, top with whipped topping
- Add blueberries to sliced strawberries, raspberries and blackberries, oranges, cherries and bananas for a fruit salad

Where to find more Information:

- *US Highbush Blueberry Council - www.blueberry.org*
- *Eat Your Blueberries - http://diet.ivillage.com*

Portion Control

It may be a problem that you have only when out and about. It may be brought on by social situations, or maybe it happens when you are bored and all alone. That's right, I'm talking about over-eating. If you grew up having to clear your plate, then this can be a huge problem when dining out. Restaurant portion sizes, especially in the United States, are one of the many problems facing those individuals trying to watch their caloric intake. Many of us eat whatever is put in front of us. After the meal, we look at the damage and cringe at the thought of what we really did to ourselves.

Amy Mac's Hints...

Avoiding "Point of No Return" Moments:

• Sometimes a restaurant will let you order off of the kids menu or even the lunch menu at dinner time.

• Ask for a to-go box to be delivered when your food is served, then put half of it in the box and proceed to clear your plate. This is one of my favorite tips because not only does it save you calories from that meal, but you also have a great leftover lunch for the next day.

Nuts

Nuts had a bad reputation for a long time because they're high in calories and fat. After years of research, it turns out that these guys aren't so bad after all. Although they're still high in calories, they bring so much good stuff with them that it is worth the calorie sacrifice. They're helpful in lowering cholesterol, preventing the hardening of the arteries and reduce your risk of heart disease. Portion control is essential when eating nuts, though, because of all the calories. Studies have shown that eating one ounce per day is all you need to see the benefits. You also need to focus on eating the nuts that are not salted or fried in oil. There is also research that found that since nuts are high in fat and fiber, they are filling and could be helpful when losing weight. There are lots of ways to incorporate nuts into your diet.

Add Them To:

- Yogurt
- Stir Fry
- Trail Mix
- Salad

Where to find more Information:

- *Nuts: good for your heart - www.clevelandclinic.org*
- *It's Full of Fat and Helps You Lose Weight - www.onhealth.com*
- *Benefits of Eating Nuts - www.health.harvard.edu*

Bulking Up

One of the most common concerns from women I train is that they are worried about bulking up. I'm quick to reassure them that women do not have the hormones present in their body to bulk up. The next concern is that they have lifted weights before and it DID make them bigger. How is this possible? The answer is simple: Building muscle is just that - building muscle. Despite its calorie-burning qualities, it does not automatically make the fatty tissue go away. Even though muscle is denser than fat, it is underneath the fat. So no matter how great your muscles may look, the layer of fat is covering it all up! The best way to remedy this is to make sure your workout routine has enough cardio in it to burn up calories, which will, in turn, reveal those muscles and create a leaner, tighter physique. Muscle does burn more calories than fat, but it may not be enough to cause weight loss on its own. A balanced resistance and cardio routine will ensure that your body is building the desired lean body mass.

Where to find more Information:

- *Benefits of Lifting Weight for Women - www.associatedcontent.com*
- *Strength Training for Women - www.trulyhuge.com*

Fresh vs. Frozen

There is rarely a nutritional difference between fresh and frozen fruits and vegetables. If anything, the frozen may be better for you because it's picked and then frozen immediately after. Anything you buy in the produce aisle is picked and then shipped to the store, possibly losing a little bit of its nutritional goodness. Overall, the decision is up to you. You may find that buying frozen is more convenient because it won't go bad right away, and you can have your favorites all year long. On the other hand, you may be too impatient to wait for those strawberries to thaw so fresh may be a better option. The one thing to keep in mind when choosing frozen; make sure it's not mixed with a sugary syrup. You also want to watch the sodium levels. Either way, rest easy because whether you prefer fresh or frozen you're still going to have the healthy benefits of fruits and vegetables.

Where to find more Information:

- *Fresh Vs. Frozen - www.stayinginshape.com*
- *Which is Best? Canned, Frozen or Fresh? - www.ext.colostate.edu*
- *Sodium: Are you getting too much? - www.mayoclinic.com*

Diet Soda

Studies show that those who consume diet soft drinks are more likely to be overweight with every can they drink. This is due to the fact that the sugar substitute leads the body to craving more sweet stuff - stuff with calories! Those who give in to those cravings are ruining the whole point of drinking diet. Just switching from regular to diet is not an effective weight loss plan. If it's part of an overall change in food selection, then switching to diet soda may be helpful. Some people find that drinking diet soda helps to add a little flavor to their otherwise bland diets. Others are so addicted to their daily soda that going cold turkey is just not possible. Whatever your reasoning, keep in mind that diet sodas may not be the miracle you're looking for.

Where to find more Information:

- *Drink More Diet Soda, Gain More Weight? - www.webmd.com*

Midnight Snacking

Is a midnight snack really that bad? The answer is no. You can have a snack later in the evening if you have not exceeded your calorie allowance for the day. Although, you may try to choose your snack wisely so you don't eat too many calories. You also need to watch the portions so as not to overeat. You don't want to go to sleep on a full stomach. Don't let your guard down just because it's late - if you have watched your calories throughout the day, don't ruin it before bed.

Amy Mac's Hints...

Good Snacking Choices:
- Veggies
- Fruits
- Cereal
- Sugar Free, Fat Free Instant Pudding

Where to find more Information:

- *Midnight Snack Won't Pack Fat - www.webmd.com*
- *Avoiding Weight Gain by Putting Late-Night Hunger to Rest*
  - http://preventdisease.com

Cardio or Weights, Which is First?

We're all looking to maximize our workouts and burn the most calories. I am often asked which should be done first, cardio or weights? It doesn't matter which is first, it matters that you do both. So if you hate cardio, are you really going to do it after you've lifted, you're tired, hungry and want to go home? No, you will either skip it or shorten that part of your workout. The same is true if you don't enjoy resistance training. I have had great success with my clients when they look forward to the second part of their workout. It sometimes makes them work harder on the first half so they can get through it and move to the second half. The only thing is to make sure you warm up if you want to lift first. Do a 5-10 minute cardio warm up, move on to weight lifting, then go back and finish the cardio portion. There are different schools of thought for each being first but if you are just looking for general weight loss and fitness, do what works for you!

What is a Fruit and Veggie Serving Size?

We all know that we should eat five servings a day of fruits and vegetables. The question is: What counts as a serving? After a little bit of research, I have found that reaching five servings a day shouldn't be that difficult. You can get a serving from any of the following:

- A medium sized piece of fruit
- 1⁄2 cup raw, cooked, frozen or canned fruits or vegetables, but it has to be in its own juice
- 3⁄4 cup of 100% juice
- 1 cup of leafy greens or 1⁄4 cup dried fruit

If you are extremely active and have a high calorie diet, you need to eat seven to nine servings of fruits and vegetables instead of the recommended five. Make sure the products you consume are low in sodium and don't have added sugar. There are lots of ways to incorporate fruits and vegetables into your diet, so be open-minded and creative.

Where to find more Information:

- *What's A Serving - www.5aday.com*

Stressed & Overworked? You need Exercise!

We all know that exercise is important. We also know that when we're stressed we need it the most. But who can find the time to take time off and go to the gym when they're already overworked and under pressure? Statistics show that walking away from the source of stress to workout, or eat a healthy meal, actually makes you more productive. It's very important to keep that blood flowing - that's what feeds the brain. Have you ever stared at something so long that you zoned out? This is actually caused by your inactive behavior. Try to take a five-minute break every hour. Stand up, walk around, stretch, pour another glass of water and return to your project refreshed.

Where to find more Information:

- *Stress: The Hidden Factor For Weight Gain - www.newhope.com*
- *Managing Stress with Regular Exercise - www.mindtools.com*

Under Stress and Overweight

Weight gain has always been a side effect of stress, usually because of the over-eating or intake of junk food during stressful times. Recent research shows that the hormone cortisol escalates in stressful times and settles in your mid-section. No need to panic though; exercise is a proven cure. Don't forget - eating healthy and trying to keep your exercise routine is crucial in times of stress. Even if you shorten your workout, something is better than nothing. Also keep in mind, your blood sugar needs to be regulated to keep you from that mid-afternoon slump. The lesson: Keep moving, eat sensibly and meet that deadline!

Where to find more Information:

- *Stress: The Hidden Factor For Weight Gain - www.newhope.com*
- *Managing Stress with Regular Exercise - www.mindtools.com*

Stretching

You know that you should stretch each time you workout. But do you know why or how to do it correctly? Stretching has many benefits, among them are flexibility, increased circulation, better posture and improved coordination. All of these things are necessary in your overall health and fitness goal. The most common stretching mistake is that people stretch before warming up. If you are one of these people, stop that habit right now! Cold stretching can result in pulled muscles! You need to warm up with low intensity cardio for 5-10 minutes before you begin stretching or doing any high intensity activity. Stretches should be held for 30 seconds each. Make sure you are not bouncing and that you are breathing.

Where to find more Information:

- *Stretching: Focus on flexibility - www.mayoclinic.com*
- *Importance of stretching often ignored - http://the.honoluluadvertiser.com*

Healthy Chocolate

It's about time someone found a healthy outlook on chocolate. Now, keep in mind, this doesn't allow you to eat tons of it all the time, but studies have shown that dark chocolate has some health benefits. Dark chocolate, and dark chocolate only, contains antioxidants that help rid your body of free radicals. It has also been proven to help you lower blood pressure. Important note: If you follow that chocolate bar with a glass of milk, you have cancelled out any good it may have done. Milk actually hinders the absorption of antioxidants. As always, remember that moderation is the key, and any calories spent on chocolate have to be left out somewhere else.

Where to find more Information:

- *Dark Chocolate is Healthy Chocolate - www.webmd.com*
- *Chocolate 'has health benefits' - http://news.bbc.co.uk*

Posture

Proper posture has a huge effect on more than just beauty pageant queens. It can help prevent neck and back problems, keep your blood circulating correctly and portray a bit of self-confidence. It is important to sit tall, pull your shoulders down and back, keep your chest high and make sure your hips are not tilted forward or backward. At first, these steps will seem unnatural and tiresome, but in actuality - training your body to do this will bring a lifetime of safety and stability to your spine and muscular system.

Make it a goal this week to work on these 4 steps toward improving posture.

1. Sit tall
2. Shoulders down and back
3. Chest high
4. Hips in neutral position

It only takes a minute to re-align yourself, take a deep breath and get back to work.

Where to find more Information:

- *Posture for a Healthy Back - www.clevelandclinic.org*
- *The Posture of Success - www.healthandwellnessclub.com*

Warm Up & Cool Down

No matter how slow and boring they may seem, the warm-up and cool-down are essential parts of your workout. Warming up is valuable because it increases the blood flow and allows your muscles and cardiovascular system to adapt to increased demands. It is much like warming up a car in cold weather - it just makes everything run a little smoother. Warming up and cooling down are both essential for healthy, happy muscles. Sudden starts or stops are literally a jolt to the system. Be nice to your body, it has been working hard! The cool-down is a great way to slow your heart rate and begin the recovery process. In addition, this is a great time to stretch. Your muscles are warm so you can concentrate on flexibility. In addition, the cool-down and stretching are important to keep your body from getting sore and tight after a workout. So spend an extra few minutes warming up, cooling down and stretching. It will enhance your workout results.

Amy Mac's Hints...

Warming Up & Cooling Down Tips:
- Start with small motions before moving up to big!
- Walk before and after you run!

Where to find more Information:

- *Warm Up Exercises - www.pponline.co.uk*
- *Adjust to Your Workout - www.mayoclinic.com*

Laughter

We've all heard that laughter is the best medicine. After a little bit of research, I can honestly say that this is one powerful reaction! Several studies have actually proven how good laughter is for you. Some of the following is what my research found.

1. Keep a hearty laugh up for 15 minutes, you could burn anywhere from 10-40 calories!

2. People that have a good sense of humor and laugh more often are less likely to have a heart attack.

3. Laughing works your abs, chest, shoulder and back muscles, just to name a few! Big laughs, big workout!

4. In addition, there's the mental health and stress reducing benefits. Have you ever had that "I'm either going to laugh or cry" moment? Next time try laughing. It is good for your heart, and you might lose a pound while you are at it.

Where to find more Information:

- *Is Laughter the Best Medicine? - www.bupa.co.uk*
- *Laughter is the Best Medicine for Your Heart - www.umm.edu*
- *Burning Calories a Laughing Matter? - www.diabetesselfmanagement.com*

Tea

It seems like everything you see has green tea in it. You can buy every type imaginable. The question is: Which one is best? First off, let me tell you that tea really does have amazing benefits. There is real proof that the powerful antioxidants in tea can help fight cancer, cavities, high cholesterol and more. In addition, it has the caffeine boost that some of us need in the afternoon. The next dilemma: Which tea to pick? Green tea is the one with all the hype, but what about black, white and other lesser-known teas? Do they have the same effect? The answer is yes. They all contain the antioxidants, but the white and green teas are more potent because of their preparation process. While black tea is not as potent, the benefits are still aplenty and it may have other benefits due to its own preparation process. Make sure to check out my links for an in-depth explanation on the differences. The next question is: Should I drink iced or hot? It's up to you: The health benefits are the same as long as the iced tea is brewed, not instant. There is so much more to cover on this topic that we'll come back to it at a later time. In the meantime, drink tea! You will be healthier if you drink as little as one cup and as many as eight cups.

Where to find more Information:

- *Time for Tea - www.youmeworks.com*
- *Wild About White Tea - http://chinesefood.about.com*
- *The Miracle of Green Tea - http://chinesefood.about.com*
- *Green Tea Can Block Cancer - http://news.bbc.co.uk*

Vitamin Fortified Water

So now it appears that regular 'ole water just isn't good enough anymore. Now it has to be pimped out with vitamins, minerals and anything else you can think of- including calories! Don't be fooled by this marketing ploy. This beverage is not only pricey but also calorie-filled. Maybe I'm alone on this one, but I don't want to spend 150 calories on a bottle of water! On some reviews, some of these waters didn't even contain what their labels claimed. The whole thing is just a little shady, if you ask me. If you are in love with these drinks, take a minute and read the label before you chug it down. How many calories is it going to cost you? Keep in mind that you have to check the serving size, because I would be willing to bet it isn't the whole bottle! Don't forget how much that beverage cost your wallet. I bet you it's more than a glass filled from the tap. And last: Does it deliver all the energy, endurance and strength that it promised? Well, nonetheless, I try to keep this informative and unbiased, but I think you all know where I stand on this one. I think a daily vitamin is a great thing, but take a pill and wash it down with plain boring water!

Where to find more Information:

- *Bottled Water is Still Pure, But It's Not Simple Anymore - http://nytimes.com*
- *Glaceau Vitamin Water Review - www.bevnet.com*

Heat Exhaustion

When the summer heat is bearing down, it's a good time to think about keeping yourself healthy in hot temperatures. First and foremost, stay hydrated! You know that drinking water is important, but when it is hot and you are sweating you are in need of more fluids than usual. Remember that if you're thirsty, your brain is telling you it needs water! If you're planning on exercising or spending lots of time in the sun, keep these symptoms in mind: headache, dizziness, light-headedness, fatigue and vomiting. Also, keep in mind any medications you may be taking because antihistamines, beta-blockers and diuretics will all increase your chance of dehydration. Some preventative measures include wearing light-colored, loose-fitting clothes. Try to plan activities in the shade or later in the day when it has cooled down a bit. Being mindful of how you're feeling is crucial to recognizing early symptoms. Be smart and enjoy your summer sun!

Amy Mac's Hints...

Preventative Measures:

- Drink lots of water
- Be aware of symptoms
- Wear light-colored, loose clothing
- Find shade if the sun is beating down

Where to find more Information:

- *Heat Exhaustion and Heat Stroke - www.emedicine.com*
- *Heat Stroke: First Aid - www.mayoclinic.com*

It's A Little "Fishy"

Lately, the government has been giving warnings about eating fish. I don't know about you, but I can never remember the ones that I'm suppose to eat. So I just don't eat any of them. This is the same mentality that lots of Americans have taken in the last couple of years. This means that we are missing out on a great source of omega-3 and protein. It is reportedly good for your eyes, brain and heart, not to mention the fact that most fish are low in calories and fat. And for those of you watching your weight, that is very important. According to the "experts," you can consume up to 12 ounces of fish per week, and this is fish of reasonable mercury content. That means no more shark dinners! You can, however, enjoy tilapia, trout, shrimp and light canned tuna (which is better for you than white canned tuna.) The mercury content is higher in the bigger, older fish because they eat the smaller fish that contain the mercury as well, thus causing a chain reaction in the predators. The main thing to remember is that moderation is the key. You can and should eat some fish because of the health benefits. But overdoing it, just like anything else, can cause problems.

Amy Mac's Hints...

Fish You Should Enjoy:
- Tilapia
- Trout
- Shrimp
- Light Canned Tuna

Where to find more Information:
- *Eating Fish: There's a Catch - www.usatoday.com*
- *What You Need to Know About Mercury in Fish and Shellfish*
  - www.epa.gov

Movie Blockbusters Making You Fat

I'm sure you've noticed all the great movies in the theaters lately. Have you thought about how dangerous the theater could be for your waistline? How about if I tell you that a large popcorn has approximately 1500 calories, and that is without the extra butter. Don't forget the soda at 100 calories per 8 ounces. Now you are looking at 400 calories. That brings the total close to 2000 calories for your movie snack! That is more calories than some people need in an entire day. If you add candy, oh boy, those are all over-sized. Some have three or four times the usual container. We aren't even going to get into the calorie content on those. My recommendation is to eat before you go to the movies. If you have to have popcorn, split the kid's size with a friend.

Where to find more Information:

- *Academy-Award-Winning Movie Snacks - www.webmd.com*
- *Counting Calories in Drinks, Juices 'n Beverages - www.dietbites.com*
- *Fixing a Fat Nation - www.washingtonmonthly.com*

Calcium - A Good Friend

We all know that calcium is important for strong healthy bones, especially in older women. But, it turns out calcium does a lot more than you may be aware of. It helps keep teeth healthy, it can help prevent colon cancer, may enhance weight loss and make your heart healthier. It's best to receive calcium through foods such as fortified juice, low-fat yogurt, milk, tofu and sesame seeds. However, if you need to take a calcium supplement, there are a couple of rules to follow. Do not take a dose of more than 500 mg at one time. Smoking, too much caffeine and sodium can reduce calcium absorption. The most commonly found supplement is calcium carbonate, and you need to take it with food. You will increase absorption if you take it with vitamin D, and also if you take it at night. Remember not to overdo the dose because too much calcium can lead to kidney stones. Also, if you take medication for hypothyroidism, you need to take the calcium 4 hours before or after to avoid affecting the thyroid medication absorption.

Where to find more Information:

- *Hypothyroidism: Can calcium supplements interfere with treatment? - www.mayoclinic.com*
- *The Surprising Benefits of Calcium - www.findarticles.com*

Notes

Use the following section to keep notes of things you would like to
accomplish, tips you found interesting or comments you would like
to send back to Amy Mac at www.withamymac.com.

Tips 26-50

Fitness Attack

No More Side Bends

I see you do it at the gym, and I hear you asking me the same question, so here is the answer: Stop doing the weighted side bends. This is where you hold a dumbbell and then lean to one side while facing forward and then stand back up. It is not going to make your love handles smaller. Think about it - you lift weights to make your muscles bigger and stronger, right? Then why would you want that for your waist? This same logic goes for females as well. Plus, if you want to get technical, your obliques are designed for the twisting motion so doing side bends isn't going to effectively work them anyway. Try doing rotating crunches, this is where you do a small crunch to one side, come back to center and then crunch to the other side. I know there are a lot of sources out there that recommend you do side bends, so don't take my word for it. Check out my resources and do your own research for an alternate move.

Where to find more Information:

- *Waist Whittling - www.fitlinxx.com*
- *Lose Your Love Handles in 3 Moves - http://fitnessmagazine.com*
- *Obliques With A Twist - http://fitnessmagazine.com*
- *The Best Tested Ab Moves Workout - www.shape.com*

Breakfast

Your mom said it, your roommate said it, the TV said it, and now I'm saying it - breakfast is the most important meal of the day. It really does set the tone for the rest of your day both in nutrition and energy. It's been proven that kids and adults do better throughout the day after a healthy breakfast. It also starts up your metabolism and gives you energy. Plus, if you have a hearty breakfast, you are less likely to overeat at lunchtime. In addition, when you make a healthy breakfast choice, you tend to keep with that trend for your other meals. There's no excuse for skipping this meal. If you're always running late, grab a whole grain English muffin with some peanut butter on it, or maybe some yogurt. It's fast, easy and portable! If you have a little more time, enjoy some oatmeal or eggs. It's a fact that one of the most important steps in losing weight is to eat a good breakfast. No more excuses, start your day off right!

Where to find more Information:

- *Break Away for Breakfast: Don't opt out of this beneficial meal - www.mayoclinic.com*
- *The Importance of Breakfast - www.intelihealth.com*
- *Breakfast is for Weight Loss Champions - http://weightloss.about.com*

Music for Your Health

Music is good for your mind, your mood and even your aches and pains. It's becoming more common to incorporate music therapy for people suffering depression, anxiety, cancer, high blood pressure and even those with attention deficit disorders. Soothing, happy tunes can improve your spirits, your outlook and your blood pressure, but the opposite is true as well. Sounds you dislike or associate with anger, anxiety or stress can arouse those negative feelings, as well. There have also been some studies that indicate listening to Mozart can even make you smarter. Fun fact: Statistics have shown that those individuals with some type of music education are less likely to have trouble with the law than those who don't.

Where to find more Information:
- *Music Therapy: How and Why is it Effective? - http://stress.about.com*
- *The sounds of music: music can have remarkable benefits for your health or it can be destructive - http://findarticles.com*

Cheating the "Regular Soda" System!

You can't give up the soda but don't want the calories, sugar or carbs. What now? I'll give you sodaholics some advice. A bottle of regular soda has 250 calories and a bottle of diet has 0. So if you're looking to cut some calories, the logical answer would be to switch from regular to diet. The catch: Not everyone can stand the taste of diet soda. If you can't give up soda and are looking for a compromise, allow yourself to have a soda at a place that offers a self-serve fountain machine. Then, fill your cup 1/3-1/2 with regular soda and the rest with diet. This helps with the taste issue and cuts your calories at the same time. My mom does this, and although I poke jokes as she bounces from the regular to the diet spouts, it is effective. Remember, the more diet, the fewer calories! Another thought: Add a splash of regular soda with cherry to your diet soda for a little variety and only a few calories.

Arthritis & Exercise

Exercising with arthritis was once thought impossible and impractical. These days, however, doctors send patients to personal trainers, like myself, to learn stretches, cardio progressions and basic strength exercises. I've seen, firsthand, the client's improvements in joint mobility and decrease in pain, just from working out. When you exercise, the cartilage in your joints is replenished with the necessary lubrication to prevent stiffness and decrease pain and swelling. In addition, your muscles become stronger and your cardiovascular health improves. If you're struggling with extra pounds, working out will also help you fight that battle. Check out the Mayo Clinic link to find some exercises that can increase the mobility of your hands. If you're an arthritis sufferer, make sure you talk with your doctor and pay attention to any restrictions or instructions he or she may give you specific to your condition. According to the research, exercise may be the best pain reliever yet.

Where to find more Information:

- *Exercise to Treat Arthritis - www.webmd.com*
- *Hand Exercises for Arthritis Pain Relief - www.mayoclinic.com*
- *Essential Treatment for Arthritis - http://arthritis.about.com*
- *Role of Exercise in Arthritis - www.hopkins-arthritis.som.jhmi.edu*
- *Exercise and Arthritis - www.arthritis.org*

Coffee - Our Little Wonder Drug

For those of you who can't make it through the day without a cup or two or three of coffee, I have some good news. Several studies show that the antioxidants and the caffeine in coffee are making you healthier. An average of three cups a day can help prevent Type 2 diabetes in women. As little as one cup can help prevent Parkinson's, and its diuretic effect can help prevent kidney stones. Plus, caffeine can play a role in helping you focus and be more productive. Be careful not to load up on too much - the caffeine can make you jittery. If you put sugar and cream in your coffee, it can add to a calorie bust. This advice goes for all the fancy coffee drinks, as well. Keep it simple, and keep it in moderation, because caffeine is a drug! Until I find other studies condemning coffee, I guess you are free to get your java jolt.

Where to find more Information:

- *Coffee's Perks - www.health.com*
- *Study Touts Coffee's Health Benefits - www.usatoday.com*
- *New Health Benefits for Coffee Drinkers - http://wbztv.com*
- *Coffee: Health Benefits and Risks - www.mothernature.com*
- *Coffee. The New Health Food? - http://men.webmd.com*

Low-Fat Scandal

I find that when I question clients about their food intake, I hear a lot of justification with the term low-fat. I ate several cookies, but they were low-fat, or I ate a coffeehouse muffin but it was low-fat. There are several misconceptions about this term, and I want to make all of you aware about what the low-fat scandal entails. Calories in and calories out are how you gain and lose weight. Low-fat does not play a role in this game. Sometimes, low-fat does mean lower calorie but many times it does not. Sometimes, they actually add more calories and more sugar to make up for the fat that isn't there. That's not going to help you at all! Plus, people tend to over eat low-fat foods because they think it is OK. For instance there are several cookies and candies that are a "low-fat food." Check out the package. They still have calories! What counts in the weight game is calories. Do not equate low-fat with making you less fat.

Where to find more Information:

- *Fat versus Fiction: Does a low-fat diet equal a leaner body?*
  - http://findarticles.com
- *Calorie Count Shockers - www.findarticles.com*
- *Starbucks Calories - www.healthyweightforum.org*

Smoothie Store Smackdown

Call me old fashioned, but I'm a little confused. I've seen several gyms with a smoothie shop located inside! This leads people to think that smoothies are healthy and part of your workout routine. I can't tell you how many people I see walking on the treadmill with their super sized smoothie where the water bottle should be. Take a guess how many calories are in a regular-size smoothie. I'm sorry, did you say as many as a soda? You are close... triple that number and then add sugar and carbs galore along with a couple of servings of fruit. Yes, folks, there are generally a few hundred calories in that post workout treat. So you burn 400 calories and then put them right back in before you walk out the door. Don't fall for the temptation or the trickery. I bet they are delicious, but check out the facts first. If you are craving that banana taste after your workout - eat a banana.

Spot Training

There is a common misconception on strength training. Working your inner thighs all day is not going to make them smaller. The same is true with your abs and every other muscle on your body. There is no such thing as spot training. In order to lose fat in one area you have to lose overall body fat, and your body will decide where the weight comes off first. Burning calories with a combination of cardio and strength training while watching your calorie intake will help you achieve this result. This doesn't mean that you should stop doing your current strength training exercises, it just means that no matter how great the muscle looks, it can still be hiding underneath body fat.

Where to find more Information:
- *Abs Demystified - http://exercise.about.com*
- *Can You Really 'Tone' Your Body - http://exercise.about.com*

Energy Drinks

Energy drinks are popping up everywhere and have a variety of claims. What do they really do to your body and will it really increase your performance? These drinks are not to be confused with sports drinks.

Extreme caffeinated beverages are all the craze both in the gyms and in the bars. Do you really need all that caffeine and sugar, not to mention all the extra calories? These drinks normally have caffeine equivalent to a cup of coffee (around 80 mg), which isn't usually dangerous. After researching some of the other newer drinks, I found some with "energy blends" equaling 2500 mg. for an 8 oz. serving. What bothers me is the push for you to drink this while doing an athletic activity. These drinks increase your heart rate and dehydrate your body. I'm not actually sure how much our bodies can handle, but those factors combined with a strenuous activity or alcohol seems like a recipe for disaster.

Where to find more Information:

- *Taurine Supplement Information and Benefits - www.bodybuildingforyou.com*
- *Medical experts warn on unhealthy buzz touting energy drinks*
  - http://seattletimes.nwsource.com
- *'Energy Drinks' stir health debate - www.intelihealth.com*
- *Caffeine and Energy Boosting Drugs - www.brown.edu*

Other Forms of Cardio

When you think of cardio, you think of running or gliding on the elliptical machine. If neither of those entices you, you might think that you're in trouble and destined to carry those extra pounds. That's not true at all. There are lots of options. First, if you're a gym member you can participate in lots of aerobic classes including kickboxing, Pilates, yoga, spinning or step. If you're on your own, you can walk, jump rope, rollerblade, bike or swim. One of my favorites is the rowing machine because it works your entire body. Make sure to ask for assistance before jumping on. If done improperly, you can really mess up your knees and back. It doesn't matter what you are doing as long as you are doing it! If you make it fun, you'll stick with it longer.

Amy Mac's Hints...

Think Outside the Treadmill:
- Play tennis
- Ski
- Surf
- Dance or skip!

Brushing Teeth = Less Heart Disease?

At the end of the summer, you're running around, finishing up vacations, enjoying the weather, getting ready for back-to-school time and you've really let your health and fitness regimen slip. Don't be so hard on yourself - there may be one habit that has been working in your favor. Have you been brushing your teeth? Studies show that there may be a correlation between brushing your teeth and reducing your risk for heart disease. It could be that the more bacteria in your mouth, the more inflammation in your arteries, which then reduces the blood flow. Or it could be that the sticky bacteria from your mouth are sticking to the plaque buildup in your arteries, causing increased blockage. Despite the technicalities, brushing your teeth is good for your smile, your breath and maybe even reducing heart disease and diabetes.

Where to find more Information:

- *Brush and Floss Regularly for Good Oral Health - www.deltadentalca.org*
- *Dental Care and Diabetes - www.webmd.com*
- *Periodontal Disease and Heart Health - www.webmd.com*

Power Napping

It's the middle of the afternoon, and you can't see or think straight. Either you had a liquor lunch or you are in need of a power nap. I've personally been napping for years. No matter how early I go to bed or get up, by 2:00 or 3:00 in the afternoon I shutdown. I've slept in airports, classrooms and mall parking lots. For years, my husband, mom and friends have been dealing with what they consider "my problem" and then lecture me on how I should sleep more at night. For me, that just doesn't do it. I'm beginning to read and see more and more that there are lots of people just like me. Napping has been shown to increase productivity, creativity and even just happier people! Studies have shown that 20-30 minutes is the best length for a nap because it does not allow you to slip into deep slumber, which can cause you to awake groggy. There are even companies offering sleep rooms and a company that leases a napping pod! If 20 minutes revitalizes you - that's great! You can sneak that in on a lunch break. I, however, need an hour. And after all these years, there is even some research stating that an hour will work, if you are waking between sleep cycles. We all have our quirks and knowing what works for you will increase your productivity and your mood.

Where to find more Information:

- *"Power Nap" Prevents Burnout; Morning Sleep Perfects a Skill - www.nih.gov*
- *A Place for the Power Nap - www.time.com*

Sweat to Heal

Your nose is running, your head aches and you have an awful cough. Do you still go to the gym? Are you a believer in sweating out a cold? If so, there are some things you should know. Sweating rids your body of water and sodium. Its main function is to regulate body temperature, not rid toxins from your system. There is a simple evaluation you should run through before hitting the gym. Are your symptoms above the neck (meaning stuffy nose or headache)? If they are and you don't feel rundown or nauseous, then you may workout; but slower and less intense than usual. If your symptoms are below your neck, such as a cough, chest congestion and nausea, then you need to take a day or two off and work on resting to make that cold better. If you continue with your workout routine when the symptoms are below the neck, you're taking a risk that your cold may turn into something more serious like pneumonia or bronchitis. Working out is great but there are times when your body needs to put the energy elsewhere. There are also concerns about spreading germs at the gym as well. If you do feel a cold coming on, it's always good to decide to workout at home or make sure you wipe down all your equipment at the gym.

Where to find more Information:

- *Working Out With A Cold - www.military.com*
- *Cold Remedies: What Works, What Doesn't and What Can't Hurt
  - www.mayoclinic.com*

Bingo Arms

It's every woman's fear - the day we can no longer wear tank tops or sleeveless dresses, due to the back of the arm that dangles for miles. Yes, ladies, the dreaded "bingo arms." The good news is that they are manageable, but you have to be knowledgeable about what it takes to manage them. Nearly all of my clients are craving those sculpted arms you see on celebrities. Our big mistake: not working our tricep muscles enough. If you break the names down, "bi" meaning two and "tri" meaning three, you will realize that you need to work your triceps more than your biceps because you are sculpting three instead of two heads. The tricep makes up 2/3 of the size of your arms and is located on the backside of your upper arm. Plus, this area is generally a popular location for fatty tissue, so you have to strength train hard using light-mid weights and doing 15-20 reps to fight the fat.

Amy Mac's Hints...

Optional Exercises:
- Kickbacks
- Presses
- Pull downs
- Dips
- Yoga pushups

Don't neglect the biceps; just try to be proportional when weight-training. Also, as you do your cardio and lose weight, this problem will become less obvious.

Everyday Activities Add Up

Eat less, move more. You know the mantra, but can't figure out where to add more action into your daily routine. The answer may be right under your nose. Do you wash the dishes by hand or use a dishwasher? Do you walk behind the mower or ride around the yard, working on your tan? Scrubbing the floors (by hand), making the bed, cleaning out your closet, doing laundry and more all burn calories. It may be just a few at a time, but they all add up. Have a competition with yourself to see how many extra little things you can do to create movement for yourself, and get a few little tasks done at the same time. Keep in mind that some of the things that you may be doing in your life, out of habit, could be making you fat.

Where to find more Information:

- *Calorie Burning Calculator - www.toneteen.com*
- *Key to "Low Metabolism" - and Major Factor in Obesity*
  - www.newswise.com

Fingernails: Window to What's Going on Inside?

If you have ever really examined your fingernails, you would notice they all look a little different. Some are stronger, prettier, discolored or spotted and you think, "wow, my nails look great," or "gee they look really awful." You never stop to think that they may indicate something more drastic. White nails could be a sign of liver disease. Dark lines beneath the nails could mean melanoma. Now these aren't sure-fire indicators, but keeping an eye on your nails could help you judge how you're doing with your diet or vitamin intake. You should also ask your doctor at your next check-up to take a look at your clean, unpolished nails as a proactive measure.

Where to find more Information:

- *Nails: How to Keep Your Fingernails Healthy and Strong - www.mayoclinic.com*
- *What Your Nails Say About Your Health - www.medicinenet.com*

Flaxseed: Whole, Ground or Oil?

Both whole and ground flaxseeds contain fiber and omega-3. Flaxseed oil also contains omega-3, but it doesn't have the fiber like the whole or ground. The oil also doesn't have all the anti-oxidant properties of the whole or ground. Flaxseed is suggested because it may lower your bad cholesterol, therefore helping to fight or prevent heart disease. Ground flaxseed is the most commonly recommended because it is easier to digest than the whole. One tablespoon should provide your omega-3 fatty acid recommendation for the whole day. There's some questionable proof of the effectiveness of flaxseed, so keep your eyes peeled for the next studies. However, it looks like if you're going to take it, the ground flaxseed is your best bet over the whole or oil.

Where to find more Information:

- *Flaxseed: Which is better- ground or whole? - www.mayoclinic.com*
- *Wellness Guide to Dietary Supplements: Flaxseed - www.wellnessletter.com*
- *Alternative Medicine: Flaxseed - www.healthandage.com*

Lactose Intolerance

You may have heard people say that they are lactose intolerant. What does this really mean? Aside from having to stay away from dairy products, it means that they are unable to breakdown the sugar known as lactose. Lactose is mostly found in cow's milk, ice cream and cheese. It's a sugar that needs to be broken down into galactose and glucose in order for us to digest it. Lactase is an enzyme that is necessary to break down the lactose. If lactase is missing, it results in digestive pain, cramps, bloating and worse. There are different phases of lactose intolerance. Some can't drink milk but can have ice cream. Others can have cheese but no milk or ice cream. Yogurt is another food that may be tolerated due to the "good" bacteria that helps with digestion. Each case is different but all are easy to treat. If you think this fits you, try a week or two without any dairy and see if you feel better. Then you can try to add certain foods in order to find out what you can tolerate.

Where to find more Information:
- *Lactose Intolerance - http://digestive.niddk.nih.gov*
- *Lactose Intolerance - www.healthcastle.com*

Potatoes

Potatoes are the number one vegetable crop in the world. Did you know that here in the United States, potatoes are harvested somewhere every month of the year? They are packed with goodness and sometimes have a reputation of being unhealthy because of French fries, potato chips or loaded baked potatoes. The truth is: potatoes are good for you. They contain 1/3 of your daily-recommended Vitamin C. A cup contains almost 1/4 of your recommended B6, which is used for everything from energy in athletics, preventing cancer and high blood pressure. Also, if you're looking for some fiber, potatoes are hiding it in their skin. Don't forget that potatoes may help lower your blood pressure. A cup or medium sized potato is approximately 125 calories, so if you can resist the temptation to overload it with tasty calories, you can have a great side dish, meal or snack. So eat smart and enjoy what these guys have to offer.

Where to find more Information:

- *Potatoes - www.whfoods.com*
- *Potato Health Benefits Discovered - http://news.bbc.co.uk*

Organics

Organic food is food that is grown without antibiotics, growth hormones, conventional fertilizers and pesticides. Food that is labeled 100% organic really does have to be completely organic. There is also a USDA organic sticker that certifies that a product is at least 95% organic. Keep in mind that the terms natural, free range and others that are appearing everywhere do not ensure a certain percentage or even mean organic. Organic farming is very involved and very time-consuming and, therefore, the prices of organic foods reflect this. Is it worth it? We know that conventional farming produces food that has met all standards for health and safety. Advocates for organics claim that their food is better for you and the environment. Organic food rarely has more nutrition than conventional food, but the debate is about the pesticides and antibiotics that leave a trace or residue within us. Could this be why we're becoming immune to antibiotics ourselves? Could there be some other long-term effect that we aren't aware of yet? This is a difficult choice and one that weighs heavy on your budget. I think as more people demand the organic lifestyle; there will be things that come along that make it a more affordable choice.

Where to find more Information:

- *Organically grown foods: Evaluate your options. - www.mayoclinic.com*
- *Are Organic Foods Worth the Price? - http://nutrition.about.com*
- *Diamond Organics Food Delivery - http://diamondorganics.com*
- *The Nation Covers the Wal-Martization of Organics*
  - www.organicconsumers.org

Yogurt

We often hear about good bacteria and how our bodies need it. What is it and where do we get it? Live and active cultures, known as probiotics, may be responsible for easing digestion, lowering cholesterol, reducing the risk of cancer, enhancing your immune system and reducing allergic reactions -- that's just to mention a few. Probiotics can be found in yogurt and other dairy products stating that they contain "Live and Active" cultures. These good bacteria are needed in your intestinal tract to help fight off the bad bacteria. In addition, when you take an antibiotic, it wipes out all the good and bad bacteria. So yogurt is a great way to replace the necessary "good" bacteria. To ensure that you are getting the most out of your yogurt - an 8 oz. serving of yogurt should only be 100 calories. So be sure to compare calories, as well as fat and sugar, in whatever brand you buy. Avoid yogurts with the phrase "heat treated after culturing" because this indicates a process that can destroy the live cultures. Yogurt is also a great source for calcium, protein and vitamins. It has even been featured in some dairy weight-loss studies. In short, find a flavor you like and stock up on this valuable low-cal snack!

Where to find more Information:

- *Health benefits of taking probiotics - www.health.harvard.edu*
- *Benefits of Probiotics (Active Culture) in Yogurt - www.healthcastle.com*
- *Newer Knowledge of Dairy Food - www.nationaldairycouncil.org*
- *French Women's Diet Secret: Yogurt - www.webmd.com*
- *AboutYogurt.com - http://aboutyogurt.com*
- *Yogurt May Help Burn Fat, Promote Weight Loss - www.webmd.com*

FIT TIP #47

Vitamin C

Is Vitamin C really the cure for the common cold? Vitamin C has been through the ringer when it comes to studies on curing a cold and other viruses. Although we aren't thrilled with the results, it seems that this vitamin may fall short of our expectations. When Vitamin C is taken before you get sick, it may help reduce some of the symptoms and shorten the length of the cold. There is no obvious evidence that even large doses will cure your cold. Although Vitamin C does have its benefits, it is a great antioxidant, it helps to fight infections and it is also needed in the production of collagen (which helps to prevent wrinkles). Maxing out your intake on Vitamin C is very easy if taking a multivitamin and eating foods such as fruits/citrus juices, berries, green and red peppers, tomatoes, broccoli and spinach. There are even some cereals that are fortified with Vitamin C. It may not cure the common cold but we'll keep it around.

Where to find more Information:

- *Vitamin C and colds - www.usnews.com*
- *Nutritional Benefits of Eating Berries - http://nutrition.about.com*

Ankle Weights

We are sometimes so desperate to burn a few more calories that we'll do something that causes more harm than good. For instance, using ankle and/or wrist weights when you walk or run. It may seem like a good idea, but it causes you to walk or run unnaturally and therefore may increase your chances of a strain or other injury. You are much better off to walk faster, longer or both. The weights only increase your calorie burn by about five calories per mile. To compensate, you can move a little faster, incorporate a short resistance routine at the end of your workout or learn proper techniques to maximize your form, which in turn will burn those additional calories. If you are looking for an alternate to the wrist or ankle weights, you can always try a weighted vest for the resistance with the least amount of strain on your arms or legs.

FIT TIP #49

Where to find more Information:

- *Walking and Weight Control - www.about.com*
- *Before You Buy Walking Weights - www.walking.about.com*
- *Fitness Quiz - www.mayoclinic.com*
- *10 Walking Mistakes to Avoid - www.walking.about.com*

Pets

Your furry friend may be helping to keep you healthy. Pets are great companions. They're also capable of providing needed stress relief, lower blood pressure, exercise and improving your mood. There have been many studies about pets and their positive effect on us. They are also so powerful that some hospitals and nursing homes are allowing dogs to visit because they're so therapeutic. It's not just the furry animals that are good. Have you ever been to a doctor's office with an aquarium? Although fish may not provide the love of a puppy, they do have a soothing effect. This pet phenomenon has even gone as far as hotels loaning you a fish for your stay. If you have the time, you may find that a pet is your best friend with a healthy bonus.

Where to find more Information:

- *Pets curb dangerous rises in blood pressure - www.cnn.com*
- *Health Benefits of Aquarium Fish - www.about.com*
- *How Owning a Dog or Cat Can Reduce Stress - www.about.com*

Notes

Use the following section to keep notes of things you would like to accomplish, tips you found interesting or comments you would like to send back to Amy Mac at www.withamymac.com.

_____

_____

_____

_____

_____

_____

_____

_____

_____

_____

_____

_____

_____

_____

Tips 51-75

Fitness Attack

Eggs

Are they good for you? Should you be eating them? What about the cholesterol?

Eggs are good for you. They're high in protein, less than 100 calories each, and aren't high in fat. They do, however, have almost a day's worth of cholesterol in them. We all know that diets high in cholesterol lead to heart problems, but we don't know how much our diets really affect our overall blood cholesterol. All sources seem to agree that eggs have some amazing healthy components. However, the large amount of cholesterol is a concern. So, for now, moderation is the key. It's okay to eat eggs, but don't go crazy especially if you have high cholesterol. When a recipe calls for eggs, use egg whites rather than the yolks. This will reduce the cholesterol and calories in your recipe.

Where to find more Information:

- *Eggs: Dietary Friend or Foe? - www.webmd.com*
- *Eggs: Are they good or bad for my cholesterol? - www.mayo.com*
- *Healthy Eggs - www.britegg.co.uk*
- *Weight Loss and a Healthy Breakfast - www.health.harvard.edu*

Shin Splints

Shin splints is a general term used to describe the intense pain at the front of the shin. Usually this pain is the irritation of the tissue that attaches the muscle fibers to the tibia (large bone in your lower leg). This is usually the result of exercising. It can be triggered by a change in speed, distance, incline or doing any exercise on a hard surface over a long period of time. It does demand that you rest and, if ignored, it can result in a stress fracture. Rest and ice are usually your best bet for treatment. You can also stretch your calf and eventually work on strengthening the calf muscles to prevent this injury in the future.

Where to find more Information:

- *Shin Splints - www.mayo.com*
- *Treating and Preventing Shin Splints - www.webmd.com*
- *Shin Splints - www.about.com*
- *Shin Splints - www.sportsinjuryclinic.net*

All About the Numbers

For some reason we have this compulsion to weigh ourselves on every scale we see and obsess about the result. The biggest concern we have when losing weight is just that - losing weight. To top it off, we actually believe what every scale in town tells us.

First Things First:

1. Stop weighing yourself on multiple scales. No good will come from it. Every scale is calibrated differently and they will never match up.

2. Pick one scale and weigh at the same time every day, week, month whatever you prefer. I weigh at the gym in the morning before my workout because if I have a scale at home, I obsess and weigh every time I walk by it.

3. The best time to weigh is in the morning before you eat. It's the most accurate.

Second Option:

Don't weigh at all. When working out you are losing fat and gaining muscle so your weight will fluctuate.

My Solution:

Pick a pair of pants that are a little too tight. Try them on once a week until they fit. Now, you know that you have lost inches and who cares about what the scale says! Your pants fit!

Wine: The Good, Bad and Ugly

We hear conflicting reports on wine. Should we drink a glass everyday or once a week? Is it good for my heart? Is it too high in calories?

Studies have shown that drinking one glass of wine a day can reduce your bad cholesterol, improve your good cholesterol and reduce blood clotting due to its antioxidants. Cabernet Sauvignon is usually the wine with the most of these antioxidants, called flavonoids. Like everything, moderation is the key. Nothing good comes from drinking too much, and a glass of wine generally has about 130 calories. If you like the taste of wine but are watching your calories, have half a glass of wine and fill the rest with club soda. This will cut the calories in half but keep the overall flavor of the wine.

Where to find more Information:
- *Red Wine - Yale - www.ynhh.org*
- *Diet Could Explain Health Benefits from Wine - www.staffnurse.com*
- *Red Wine - Heart Health Benefits? - www.healthcastle.com*

Sciatica

Sciatica is the shooting pain that starts in your back or butt and moves down the back of your leg into your feet. It is generally found in people 30-50 years of age and is not genetic. Sciatica, in fact, is the symptom and not the problem. It's a sign of irritation of the sciatic nerve. This can result from a herniated disc, pinched nerve or other injuries. You may sometimes experience tingling, numbness or weakness in the leg. Symptoms normally subside in a few days to a few weeks. Ice, rest, walking and ibuprofen can help reduce pain and inflammation. If this sounds like you, see a doctor for a proper diagnosis.

Where to find more Information:

- *Sciatica - www.mayoclinic.com*
- *Sciatica.org*
- *What you need to know about sciatica - www.spine-health.com*

Side Dishes Become Dinner Dishes

This may seem so remedial that you're going to dismiss this idea, but give me a minute. Using smaller plates decreases your calorie intake and, yet, fully satisfies your hunger. Think about it - if you put average or small portions on a dinner plate it just isn't the same. No heaping pile of pasta, no giant baked potato - it's missing something and you're disappointed from the start. Now put those same portions on a side plate. It looks like a ton of food, and you can eat the whole thing! Forget putting ice cream in a cereal bowl - it now goes in a ramekin, small coffee cup or a small bowl. You laugh because this is so simple and yet it's a matter of tricking your mind and stomach into enjoying what you can have instead of pining for what you can't, or shouldn't, devour. If you don't believe me, try it for a week. Use the food's single serving size and pile it onto a small plate. You'll be amazed at how much less you are eating and how guilt-free you are to clear your plate.

If the Shoe Fits

Buying shoes for exercise is a major project, but it's worth the time. Buying the wrong shoes can make your workout life miserable. The wrong fit can make you prone to injury. Your toenails can become infected making you very uncomfortable.

1. The first key to proper fitting is to wear your workout socks when shopping and trying on the shoes.

2. The next step is to shop for shoes in the afternoon when your feet are already slightly swollen.

3. Third, you want to match the shoe to the sport. Shoes are built for certain sports and have certain features. Most of these are to enhance comfort. The curve of the shoe, the weight of the sole and the flexibility are all sport specific, so take advantage.

4. Finally, don't believe all the hype over the shoe's bells and whistles. They won't do you any good if the shoe doesn't fit.

Last tip - There should be no need to "break in" the shoes. If they are not comfortable when you are wearing them around the store, they are not the shoes for you.

Where to find more Information:

- *Athletic Shoes- The Right Ones - www.uihealthcare.com*
- *Before You Buy Walking Shoes - www.about.com*
- *Wearing the Wrong Shoes - www.about.com*
- *If the Running Shoes Fits, Wear It - www.webmd.com*

Plateau

If you've ever worked out, you've probably encountered a plateau in your training. This is where you're no longer seeing results with the routine that once worked. The keyword in that sentence is routine. In order to keep your body responding, you need to keep it guessing. It doesn't always have to be drastic "over the top" changes. The first thing to try after making sure you are increasing weight, as necessary, is changing the order of the exercises. Something this simple can jumpstart your engine back up. The next thing to try is changing the frequency of your workouts. You can add or take away a workout during your week and change the intensity in which you perform it. As you become stronger you are going to have to workout harder but not all the time. Sometimes an hour walk is better than a 30 minute jog. Change the time that you devote to that exercise by adding 5 minutes to each session, or change the type of exercise you are doing. This is especially true for cardio. Make sure you mix up the cardio so your muscles and cardiovascular system don't become too comfortable with one type of exercise. You can do any of these things to break your plateau.

Where to find more Information:

- *Jumpstart your regular workout - www.ivillage.co.uk*
- *Break Your Plateau Cycle - www.askmen.com*
- *Understanding Weight Loss Plateaus - www.about.com*

Switching Equipment

We've talked about changing your routine to defeat a plateau. Now, I want to focus on another form of change -- equipment. If you always use the same things to work the same muscles, then your muscles are probably as bored as you are. Take advantage of all the products out there that allow you to enhance your workout. The stability ball is my favorite. Those are the inflated balls that you probably see at the gym and on television. There are tons of exercises to do on this that enable you to focus on working your abs, back and butt muscles, referred to as core muscles, while working another muscle group at the same time. Squats, bicep curls, chest presses and crunches are great with the challenge of the stability ball. Even switching between free weights and machines will challenge your muscles in a new way. Don't be afraid to try something new. If you don't know how to use something, ask a trainer, consult a magazine or book, or ask a more knowledgeable friend.

Amy Mac's Hints...

Equipment to Try:

- Medicine Balls
- BOSU Balls
- Resistance Bands
- Stability Ball
- Exercise Balances Discs

Where to find more Information:

- *Medicine Ball Exercises - www.ballyfitness.com*
- *Abs, Hips & Thighs on the Ball - www.about.com*
- *Abdominal Exercises - www.net.co.uk*
- *Resistance Band Exercises - http://newsinfo.iu.edu*

Beat the Boredom

Do you avoid buying workout videos because you become bored too quickly? For those of you who have a video delivery service, I have a tip for you. Check out the selection of fitness DVDs they have and add them to your play list. Then when movies are delivered, a new workout will come with it! This eliminates the boredom factor, purchasing a DVD (and hating the workout), and you can keep it as long as you like! This could be a great time to learn Pilates or yoga at a low cost, or a chance to striptease in your living room! Have fun with the selections and look forward to what is delivered. Invite friends to join you! When workouts are new and exciting, we don't think of them as work. Have fun and use this service to your advantage.

Amy Mac's Hints...

Online Workout DVD Rentals:
- Netflix (www.netflix.com)
- Blockbuster (www.blockbuster.com)

Headaches

Why isn't a headache always the same? There are different types of headaches and each has its own set of signs and symptoms. A tension headache, which is the most common, is a whole-head, stiff, achy feeling which may even affect the neck. It's caused by tension, exhaustion, hormones, stress and more. Migraines are the constricting of the blood vessels in the head and create an awful pain, which is sometimes worse on one side of the head. This pain is sometimes accompanied by nausea, light and sound sensitivity and can last hours or days. There are also headaches, which are a result of an illness or disease. Sinus problems are an excellent example of that. Indoor and outdoor allergens can create sinus problems, which then create a headache that just won't quit. Most of these problems have medications to help relieve the pain, but always be in tune with what your head is telling you. You can even take note of each headache, its location and severity to better track and identify causes.

Where to find more Information:
- *Headache - www.medicinenet.com*
- *Headache - http://uimc.discoveryhospital.com*

Bananas

Many times this fruit is split and added to ice cream. If left alone, the banana is a healthy snack and great energy booster. A medium size banana has only 100 calories. It's a good source of potassium, which is a necessary electrolyte for your body. Potassium is needed to keep water and other minerals balanced within our bodies. It also keeps muscles from cramping. Bananas contain natural sugar, which will give you an instant energy boost. They rarely cause allergic reactions and are easily digested. Add a bit of peanut butter to make a tasty before or after workout snack, or add bananas to your morning cereal for some early morning energy.

Where to find more Information:

- *Potassium and Fitness Go Hand in Hand - www.busywomensfitness.com*
- *Eat Bananas and Live Longer - http://news.bbc.co.uk*
- *Bananas Could Prevent Strokes - http://news.bbc.co.uk*
- *Bananas - www.finetuneyou.com*

Jet Lag

If you ever travel east or west, pay attention! Jet lag feels like a hangover. You get a headache, you're tired, groggy and grumpy. It's said that a recovery day is required for each time zone crossed. If you're traveling for fun, you can miss out on an entire day or weekend by napping and moping. If you're traveling for business, this can be a very trying time because you aren't exactly on your toes.

What can you do to avoid or at least minimize jet lag?

- Stay hydrated throughout the flight and after.
- Drink lots of water, not soda or liquor on the plane. Your body needs water.
- Next, try to stretch and move about while on the plane. I know this is difficult, but it is very important especially if you have a long flight.
- When you land try to find some sun and enjoy a few re-energizing moments catching some rays.
- You also need to make sure you keep your exercise routine and begin following your destination's timetable.

This will all help you wake up refreshed tomorrow.

Where to find more Information:
- *Jet Lag, Motion Sickness and More - www.health.harvard.edu*
- *Jet Lag - www.sleepfoundation.org*

SAD

If you are solar-powered like me, you'll probably become distraught when the days start getting shorter. When daylight savings time ends, it will be dark by afternoon! There are some things that will help you endure the dark and cool months a little bit better. Number one on the list is to keep exercising! Also, either keep or create a sleeping routine. This will help your energy levels, and, of course, the cooler months mean holidays with food and stress. Keep your eating habits in line. There is no way to justify all the junk food. Try to keep stress at a minimum, be organized with plans and gifts. Also, if you think you may be a sufferer of Seasonal Affective Disorder, light therapy may help you fight the blahs.

Amy Mac's Hints...

Keep or Create Those Routines:
- Exercise
- Sleep
- Eating
- Be Organized

Where to find more Information:
- *Winter Blues: Ways to Cope - http://health.ivillage.com*
- *Seasonal Affective Disorder (SAD) - www.mayo.com*
- *Seasonal Affective Disorder (SAD) - www.uihealthcare.com*
- *Facts of Light - www.ppnf.org*

What Does 3,500 Calories Equal?

One of my biggest complaints about people losing weight is that they frequently downplay their success. When you talk about a pound or two, it seems so simple and minor. The reality is that 3,500 calories equals a pound. Yes, 3,500 calories! That's a deficit of 500 calories per day for an entire week. Sounds easy but to keep that up in order to lose 20, 30 or even 50 pounds, takes some dedication and careful planning.

The equations for men and women on how many calories you should be consuming in a day are below. This equation is an estimate. It does not apply to those who are extremely muscular or obese.

Amy Mac's Hints...

English Basal Metabolic Rate (BMR) Formula:
- **Women**: BMR = 655 + (4.35 x weight in pounds) + (4.7 x height in inches) - (4.7 x age in years)
- **Men**: BMR = 66 + (6.23 x weight in pounds) + (12.7 x height in inches) - (6.8 x ages in years)

Figure your minimum calories because being aware of that number will help you manage your daily nutrition. You might think twice about dessert or "happy hour" once you begin to have calorie awareness.

Where to find more Information:
- *Losing Weight -- Start By Counting Calories - www.fda.gov*
- *BMR Equations - www.bmi-calculator.net*

Coffee Crimes

I was intrigued to see what a difference using zero calorie sweeteners in your coffee could make. I did some math and found that if you add two sugar packets and one serving (which is one tablespoon) of flavored creamer, it adds 55 calories to your coffee! Now think about how many cups you have a day or week! It adds up fast. Now, if you substitute two packs of the zero calorie sweetener flavored or unflavored packs for the sugar packets, and add skim milk instead of creamer, it only adds 5.5 calories to your coffee! That is saving you 50 calories per cup, which is huge!

Circuit Training

Circuit training is a great way to decrease your time in the gym and yet see maximum benefits out of your workout. I run all of my sessions as circuits because we want to challenge muscles as well as the cardiovascular system. We are on a time schedule and I get bored easily. There are a couple of ways to do it.

- The first is to alternate upper and lower body strength, so first bicep curls and then squats. This eliminates the rest period, which not only allows your heart rate to decrease, but it also wastes time.

- Another option is to "superset." Depending on where you are in your conditioning, you can do bench presses and then pushups. You are working the same muscles but in a different way. This will exhaust the muscle group faster, and you aren't standing around waiting for your rest period.

- Another option is alternating strength with cardio. Your heart rate is up and you will burn those calories. You can do bicep curls and then jump rope in between sets. I usually do three different exercises in each segment and then three sets of each. So if you are doing biceps, squats and jump rope, you run through those three and then start over until you have completed three of each move.

There are a million ways to workout. Find what you like and make it your own. Little tweaks to your workout make all the difference.

Where to find more Information:

- *"The 20 Minute Workout Solution" Janet Lee, Shape, September 2006*

Freezer Section - Watch Out

When the summer ends, it feels like time to curl up in your fat-roll forgiving sweatshirt (yes, we all have one) and go into hibernation mode. Warm soups and heavier dishes will quickly replace all those fabulous light summer salads you were dying for in July. My challenge for you and for myself is to keep some of those light summery foods a part of your yearly diet, not just seasonal. Buy the fruits in the frozen section and keep enjoying all their benefits, such as being low calorie and great tasting with antioxidants. Why not have a summer salad in November? Pair it with a small, hot baked potato and you have a meal. Eat your summer salad in front of the fireplace to relive those summer heat waves. Don't curl up and let that bikini body go - because next summer will come around and then you'll regret those comfort foods. If you are going to eat warm, look for low calorie soups. Keep the bread calories to a minimum, include fruit and veggies with your meals and rely on hot tea to keep you warm. Also keep in line with your portion sizes. Eating the right amount needs to be habit so there's no splurging when you can bundle up and hide that extra five.

Deep Water Running

Deep water running is becoming its own exercise. It is commonly used in rehabilitation workouts for those recovering from knee or other injuries. It can also be incorporated into your everyday exercise routine. It's a nice relief to all those joint-pounding exercises we usually partake in and has the same benefits. All you need is a buoyancy belt and a pool. You can simulate running outside or on a treadmill by doing the same thing in the deep end. You can also do high knees, which is just bringing your knee to your chest and then switching legs repeatedly. This is a great cardio workout and if you have access to a pool, you might consider it.

Where to find more Information:
- *IDEA Fitness Journal, May 2007*
- *Benefits of Deep Water Running - www.about.com*

Do I Need a Sports Drink?

I'm often asked about the necessity of sports drinks. Sports drinks serve the purpose of re-hydrating you and replenishing your electrolytes. My general rule is that if you do more than 60 minutes of cardio or are involved in an active sport or game, you may need to turn to a sports drink that will replenish the sodium and potassium your body needs at a faster rate. Water is great for hydration but sweat is more than just water, and those elements do need to be replenished quickly in a high intensity situation. However, these drinks do contain calories, and it may not be necessary to drink the whole bottle to be restored. Be sure to check the serving size so you don't get tricked into a bundle of unnecessary calories. These drinks also provide carbohydrates, which result in a burst of energy that may be helpful in endurance events or games. Don't down these drinks just to be part of the hype, really acknowledge their purpose and use them to your benefit.

Where to find more Information:

- *Effectiveness of Sports Drinks - www.about.com*
- *Gatorade Formula & Nutrition Information - http://gatorade.com*

FIT TIP #70

Glucosamine

There have been a number of questions and claims about the effectiveness of glucosamine and its ability to rebuild joint cartilage. For years, products have been on the market claiming that they could help rebuild cartilage and, therefore, reduce the pain of osteoarthritis. Some people swear by it, others aren't seeing the same results. The new word coming in, and backed by a two-year study, gives us some idea on who glucosamine helps. It turns out that when you combine glucosamine with chondroitin, you have a much more effective result. However, the effectiveness is mainly in those who are experiencing moderate to severe knee pain. It seems that those with mild pain did not notice a significant decrease in using the glucosamine chondroitin combo, glucosamine only, chondroitin alone, or a placebo. Now doctors need to study exactly how glucosamine and chondroitin work in creating relief for these sufferers.

Where to find more Information:

- *Glucosamine and Chondroitin Sulfate - http://ww2.arthritis.org*
- *Good News for Knees - http://ww2.arthritis.org*
- *Glucosamine Supplements: Can they rebuild cartilage?*
  - www.mayoclinic.com

Quinoa

Quinoa has almost twice the fiber of pasta and brown rice. It's also a complete protein, which means that all nine essential amino acids are present. Amino acids are used to build muscle. Quinoa is also full of magnesium, which is good for your heart and has twice the protein of regular cereal grains. It's inexpensive and is found in the rice aisle at the grocery store. You cook it like pasta so it's ready in twenty minutes. It is great as a side dish in place of pasta or rice. I encourage you to give it a try. It can be made so many ways, I'm confident you can incorporate this 'superfood' into your meals.

Where to find more Information:
- *Men's Health Magazine, May 2007*
- *Quinoa - www.whfoods.com*

Breast Cancer Awareness

Every time I turn around, I hear that someone else I know has been diagnosed with some type of cancer, many with breast cancer. Maybe it's a sign that I'm getting older, maybe it's a sign of the times or maybe it's that we are being proactive in catching the symptoms early. Early diagnosis is one of the keys to surviving this battle. According to the National Breast Cancer Foundation, of the women that live to be 85, 1 in 8 will develop breast cancer. This means that this disease will heavily affect both men and women. It's obvious that women are the most at risk, but men are certainly not exempt. Family history, your diet, drinking and smoking habits are all thought to be factors in your level of risk. This just reminds us to be wise with our choices and to always be aware of our physical and mental health. Never be afraid to see a doctor if you are questioning something, and remember that self-examination and yearly exams are the best methods for early detection.

Where to find more Information:

- *National Breast Cancer Foundation, Inc. - www.nationalbreastcancer.org*
- *American Cancer Society - www.cancer.org*
- *National Cancer Institute - www.cancer.gov*

Self? Help!

We're all longing to make ourselves better - better at work, better entertainers, better hobbyists, better with time management and better at health and fitness. The list never stops. Why is it that sometimes we need outside assistance to point out our faults and then provide the solution? For instance, on numerous occasions, I have spent hours being dragged up and down the aisles of the office supply store by my husband, who is determined to organize my piles and me. I don't know, something about a cluttered desk leads to a cluttered mind or something like that. I do want to be organized. I want to change, but when the days fly by, it just doesn't always happen, or ever happen. How many times have I heard that from clients when they don't make it to the gym? I would like to believe that labels, folders and totes are going to make me the most efficient person ever but, somehow, I think it takes more than that. I think it takes desire to be better and determination to make sure you stick with your new plan until it becomes habit. Who says what is or is not the right way? My piles all have a purpose and I'm productive. So do I need this drastic change? I guess there is always room for improvement. The moral of the story is: Be open to change because it could be better and healthier than the old way, and be open to suggestions because some people see things in us that we ourselves overlook.

Cortisol

I'm sure you've all seen the numerous diet product commercials claiming that cortisol, which is a stress-produced hormone, makes you fat. These products claim that they will eliminate this hormone, thus causing you to lose weight. I decided to research this concept to prove it right or wrong. After extensive research, I'm not even sure if cortisol makes you fat. So that leads me to believe that these products are questionable. According to Mayo Clinic, the amount of cortisol produced in a stressed person is not enough to cause them to gain weight, unless they have another medical condition. Other reliable sources mention that cortisol leads to belly fat. So I have to admit that I'm confused as to whether it does or does not make you fat. In further research, I found tons of studies about monitoring the cortisol levels in stressed children and other studies claiming that there may be a link between cortisol and depression. So, my conclusion, a consistently high level of cortisol is not good. It's been linked to chronic stress that encompasses a whole lot of problems, a decrease in the mental development of children, and now depression and maybe even belly fat. Now remember, I'm not a doctor but I wanted to present some of this research because it is a popular topic.

Where to find more Information:

- *Depression May Be Linked to Cortisol - www.thecrimson.com*
- *Do cortisol blockers increase weight loss? - www.mayoclinic.com*
- *Cortisol and Stress: How to Stay Healthy - www.about.com*

Notes

Use the following section to keep notes of things you would like to accomplish, tips you found interesting or comments you would like to send back to Amy Mac at www.withamymac.com.

_____

_____

_____

_____

_____

_____

_____

_____

_____

_____

_____

_____

_____

Tips 76-101

Fitness Attack

Sucralose

Sucralose is known as an artificial sweetener and the brand name is Splenda. Recently the FDA did an update on artificial sweeteners and is upholding its original 1998 and 1999 approval of this zero calorie sweetener. There have been over a hundred studies conducted through twenty years that have proven that there is no link to cancer or any other dangerous illness or disease. Splenda starts out as sugar but goes through a complicated process to become an artificial sweetener. It is not digested so, therefore, it does not affect the blood sugar levels making it safe for diabetics and also making it the 0 calorie, 0 carb sweetener we enjoy.

Where to find more Information:

- *Are Artificial Sweeteners Safe? - www.webmd.com*
- *Artificial Sweeteners and Cancer - www.cancer.gov*
- *Sugar Substitutes - www.cfsan.fda.gov*
- *Artificial Sweeteners - www.mayoclinic.com*
- *The Truth on Artificial Sweeteners - www.webmd.com*
- *Splenda.com*

Snoring

If someone in the house is snoring, you miss out on sleep. How is that fair?

Snoring is usually more annoying than dangerous for the one that snores. However, once again health and fitness are a factor in this situation. It seems that consistent, moderate exercise such as twenty minutes, three times a week may help with reducing snoring. Also, those carrying extra weight, especially around their neck area, are more likely to snore. This means we have another motivation for eating right and exercising. If you aren't the one snoring, now would be a great time to start a couple's workout program - both of you will reap the benefits.

Where to find more Information:
- *The A to Z of Snoring - www.dailyrecord.co.uk*
- *Snoring - www.sleepfoundation.org*

Where Are Your Toes Going?

We have talked about proper posture and alignment before, but I've seen an overwhelming trend of poor posture and knee problems. Many times they are related. The next time you're walking normally, glance down and see if your toes are pointed straight out in front of you. If they turn in towards each other or out diagonally, you're doing yourself a disservice. Start focusing on placing them in a 12-6 position. It's just like a clock, so that means the toes are at 12 and the heels at 6. To see and feel the benefits of this change, make sure the turn comes from the whole leg, all the way up at your hips. Your toes should be in line with your kneecap. If you make the change at just the feet, you'll still have unnecessary pressure on your knees up to your hips and then your back. It's amazing that a simple switch can make such a huge difference.

What Have You Got To Lose?

People always want to know quick tips on how to keep fit while working nonstop. The next best thing to working out is to fidget and move as much as you can, when you can. The obvious ones are to take the stairs, not the elevator, or park your car farther from your office and walk. But there are other little things, you just have to think about it.

Other "Move More" Options:

- Going to the bathroom that is farthest away from your desk
- Fidgeting with a pen or better yet, a paperweight
- Stand up and stretch at least once an hour
- Alternate sitting & standing if your work environment allows
- When you are getting ready in the morning, do toe raises while brushing your teeth
- Jump rope while waiting for the dog to do his thing outside

I do tricep dips off of office chairs, kitchen chairs, coffee tables -- there is always something around! It's also good to practice your balance, so stand on one leg while talking on the phone or when standing in line at a store. Use what you have. It's better than nothing!

The "Yes" Compulsion

My clients, my friends and myself all have the same problem and can't find the solution. We are all "yes" people. We want to help, we want to be great at our jobs, great at our friendships, great at everything and when someone asks a favor or has an invite, we always say "yes." It seems so simple to just say "no," but I'm really starting to think that it's a compulsion. We're all worried that the world would collapse if we said no. Or worse yet, the other person would be offended if we turned them down. Or even still, that the "opportunity of a lifetime" could pass us by. Living with that pressure, that stress and that self-expectation isn't healthy and we need to make a change. I don't have a fix for this one, but I do know that being aware of it helps to remind us of our limits.

Cherry Juice

After a big workout, you wonder if there is anything that will help relieve muscle soreness. There was a study at the University of Vermont which revealed that drinking tart cherry juice might help to alleviate some of that pain. Cherry juice contains anti-inflammatory and antioxidant properties, which are responsible for this benefit. The study also mentions that it may help those with "chronic, nagging pain" and so they might want to incorporate some cherry juice into their diets.

Where to find more Information:

- *Cherry Juice To Ease Sore Muscles' Pain - www.allheadlinenews.com*

Alternate Abs

Is there another way to strengthen my abs without crunches? Yes! If you aren't a big fan of crunches, there are lots of other ways to strengthen your abs. First of all, general exercise, Pilates, yoga and squeezing your abs while working out will strengthen them.

There are non-crunch exercises as well:

1. One of my favorite oblique exercises (which are the sides of your waist) is to take a medicine ball or dumbbell and put it behind you, either held by someone else, or set on a table.

2. Then put your back to it and reach around to the right and grab it.

3. Swing all the way back around to the front and over to the left side where you can set it down behind you.

4. Now repeat, moving back and forth picking up the ball and replacing it. Don't move too fast or you'll get dizzy!

Where to find more Information:
- *Flat, Sexy Abs in Record Time - www.shape.com*
- *Love Your Love Handles in 3 Moves - www.fitnessmagazine.com*

Broccoli

More Calcium than milk, more Vitamin C than oranges, broccoli is a powerhouse veggie. There have been several studies featuring broccoli as a cancer-fighting food. Broccoli actually increases the body's production of its own cancer-fighting substance. In addition to the Vitamin C and Calcium, it contains fiber and Vitamin A, which does everything from boosting your immune system to aiding in the health of the eyes, liver, brain and more. Raw or steamed broccoli is best because they contain the most nutrients. The other members of broccoli's family, cauliflower, kale, cabbage and brussel sprouts, are all thought to be likely candidates to have these same powers. At least for now, we know the power broccoli possesses, so add it to a salad, put it on a veggie tray, or steam it and put it on a potato.

Where to find more Information:

- *Broccoli beats most other veggies in health benefits - www.cnn.com*
- *9 More foods that help you live longer - www.askmen.com*
- *Broccoli Packs Powerful Punch to Bladder Cancer Cells*
  - http://researchnews.osu.edu

Antibacterial Soap

When I go to buy soap, I instantly reach for the antibacterial kind. Why? Because according to its definition and its marketing, I think I'm buying something that is better and healthier. The truth is, I am wasting my money and could actually be causing more harm than good. First, there is no study that shows that soap with antibacterial ingredients really will prevent germs, bacteria, or illnesses. Second, the body, both adult and child need to be exposed to some germs in order to stimulate their immune system. If our system never fights, it will be weakened and therefore we will catch every cold in town. There is one thing that has been proven to be the number one germ deterrent and that is simply the act of washing your hands.

Where to find more Information:

- *The Dangers of Antibacterial Soap - www.life.ca*
- *Antibacterial soap won't cut infections - www.abc.net.au*

Heat or Ice?

Have you ever been injured and wondered whether you should ice or heat your injury?

Ice and heat are both common methods to treat or minimize the pain and swelling of an injury. Heat should be used for muscle aches, stiffness and dull pains. A sore or strained muscle needs heat because it increases the circulation to that area and relaxes the injured muscles. Ice should be used to prevent swelling. Usually when we twist or sprain something, swelling is a result and so rest, ice, compression and elevation is the best thing. Neither heat nor ice should be used excessively. Twenty minutes is your maximum before taking a thirty-minute or more rest. Too much is not a good thing, especially when icing. It can decrease the body temperature in the injured area and therefore cause more blood to rush to the area to heat it up. This results in additional swelling and bruising. When dealing with heat, be careful not to burn the skin and if possible, moist heat is best.

Where to find more Information:

- *Ice or Heat - Which Should I Apply? - www.abc.net.au*
- *Ice or Heat - www.about.com*

Olive Oil

We know that olive oil tastes good, but what are its health benefits? It appears that a tablespoon a day of extra virgin olive oil will help protect against heart disease and cancer because it's full of antioxidants. Yes, olive oil is high in calories and fat, but it is the good fat that helps your body absorb all the nutrients from your salad or pasta dish, as well as make you feel full. The word "extra" means that it has less acidity than regular virgin olive oil. Also, keep in mind that oil comes from different regions so, therefore, they will all taste a little different. You'll have to experiment to find your favorite!

Where to find more Information:
- *Shape Magazine, April 2007*
- *Cooking Oil - How to choose the best one - www.healthcastle.com*

Should I Get a Flu Shot?

When my doctor asked me if I wanted to have a flu shot, I didn't know the answer. I told him I would pass for now, but do some research. I guess I've never really thought about it before, but I've heard many rumors about flu shots and I wanted to find out the truth. I did some research and the University of Maryland had most of my answers.

Does the flu shot give you the flu?

Apparently this is a myth. The vaccination doesn't contain the virus, so therefore can't give you the flu. If you get sick right after the shot, you are either having an allergic reaction, or coincidentally, caught something else.

Is it sure to work?

The flu shot may not fully prevent you from getting the flu but if you do, your symptoms will be less severe than without.

Finally - Who needs the shot?

It seems that everyone can benefit. Although, those who are younger, older or whose immune systems are weak, will benefit the most from the flu vaccine.

Where to find more Information:

- *Flu Vaccine Facts - www.umm.edu*
- *Stanford Researcher Shows Flu Shot Benefits Outweigh Costs in Healthy Young Adults - http://med.stanford.edu*

Charley Horses

If you have ever woken up to an extreme leg cramp in the middle of the night, then you know what a charley horse is.

A charley horse is a term used to describe a severe leg cramp in your foot, calf or thigh. Many times it's caused by muscle fatigue and happens when you're working out, but there are also times when you get them while sleeping. These spasms can be a result of dehydration or a mineral deficiency such as sodium, potassium or magnesium. When the cramp begins, the best thing you can do is rub or massage the muscle to help it relax and then try to stretch it. To prevent or keep them from coming on, make sure you drink plenty of water. Eating bananas and oranges will help if you're low on potassium. Making sure you incorporate stretching into your workouts will decrease some muscle tightness. There are also some medications that can bring this on so if it's new or frequent, check with your doctor to find the cause.

Where to find more Information:

- *Charley horse: muscle cramps - www.uihealthcare.com*
- *Leg Cramp - www.about.com*
- *Shape Magazine, November 2006*

Meditation

I have to admit that when I read how to de-stress or refocus or relax, meditation is always on the list of things to try. I've always thought: This isn't me and move to the next option. However, in the last few months, much to my surprise, I've realized that I do meditate! Whenever I'm overwhelmed or feel a headache coming on, I stop, close my eyes, take a few deep breaths and try to regain composure before going back to the task at hand. This is a form of meditation. I think that all the times I crossed it off the list, I was picturing something much more extreme. I know that there are thousands of ways to meditate and what works for me may not work for someone else. But when everything falls apart at once, know when to stop what you are doing, take a deep breath and then re-enter the chaos. That breath might save you from coming unglued.

Where to find more Information:

- *Meditation: Relaxing with sustained concentration - www.mindtools.com*
- *Meditation Boosts Mood, Immune System - www.webmd.com*

FIT TIP #89

Garlic

Another 'superfood' is stepping up to the plate! Garlic is one of those foods that has multiple functions. It can help to prevent cancer, helps to fight heart disease, including high cholesterol, and it helps to fight germs. Garlic contains a substance called allicin, which is what gives garlic its stinkiness, but it's also what provides these other healthy benefits. Garlic is versatile so you can add it to most anything. The only downside is having everyone else know you ate garlic.

Where to find more Information:

- *Shape Magazine, December 2006*
- *Shape Magazine, April 2007*
- *The health benefits of garlic - www.ivillage.co.uk*

Ulcers

If you think that spicy foods and stress cause ulcers, you aren't alone. Nearly seventy percent of Americans believe this as well. However, it turns out that almost all ulcers are created by a bacteria, H. Pylori. An ulcer is an open sore or a lesion that is usually thought to be in the stomach or intestines but it can be found in other areas. An ulcer is created when this bacteria invades the mucous layer and, therefore, inflames the lining of the stomach. Although food choices and lifestyle factors aren't the major cause of ulcers, they can irritate an existing one. Since it is bacteria that cause an ulcer, it can normally be cured with an antibiotic.

Where to find more Information:

- *Peptic Ulcer - www.mayoclinic.com*
- *Digestive Disorders - www.umm.edu*

Motivational Cards

I'm always in search of motivation when it comes to working out. This is a simple way to feel super productive after a trip to the gym or a jog outside.

- Buy a stack of index cards and every week fill out a card for each workout that you would like to complete for the week.

- You can assign them for certain days or just by category, whichever way you will find them most effective.

- After you workout, throw the card away and feel productive.

- You can even have a reward for yourself if you are out of cards by the end of the week.

If you are looking for a greener idea, there are dry erase calendars and post-its that will also do the trick.

Houseplants

We know that houseplants are attractive and add a little life to a dull room, but studies are showing that plants could actually improve your health both physically and mentally. Plants make you calmer and also help to fight the winter blues. They are also recommended for your office or desk to help relieve stress. But plants can be good for more than just looks. They feed on carbon dioxide and emit oxygen, which is the opposite of what we do. So therefore, when a plant is nearby, a constant cycle of oxygen and carbon dioxide is created. NASA has done some studies that show plants actually detoxifying the air in a room.

Amy Mac's Hints...

Plants That Purify:
- Spider Plants
- Ferns
- Palms
- Ivy

The question is now, how many plants do you need to see benefits? Right now, the research is pointing toward the more the better, but my thought is that one has to be better than none!

Where to find more Information:
- *The Health Benefits of House Plants... - www.sixwise.com*
- *Boost Your Health With Houseplants - www.health.com*
- *Plants: Pros and Cons - www.aerias.org*
- *Houseplants Offer Health Benefits - http://wcco.com*

Cold Weather Precautions

If you're a diehard runner or outdoor exerciser, then the cold weather is just something you live with. If you're new to working out, you should know how to prepare for the cooler temperatures.

- First, you should dress in layers. Multiple layers will keep you warmer and will also allow you to shed a layer once you warm up.

- Next, wear a hat. Up to fifty percent of your body heat lost is lost through your head, so keep it covered!

- Third, make sure you start slow and easy. When muscles are cold they're more prone to injury, so gradually warming them up eases them into the exercise and reduces the risk.

- You also need to be especially careful of your environment. Ice, snow and rain are all obstacles so be aware.

- Also, daylight disappears pretty early these days so make sure you are visible and in a safe area. If none of this sounds appealing to you, then join a gym or try some exercises at home or with videos.

Where to find more Information:
- *Layer-Up For Your Winter Workout - http://cbs5.com*
- *Cold Weather Exercise Safety - www.about.com*
- *Exercise and cold weather: Stay motivated, fit and safe*
  - www.mayoclinic.com

Childhood Obesity

According to the American Obesity Association, thirty percent of children and adolescents are overweight and fifteen percent are obese. These numbers have increased dramatically in the last few decades. In the early 1970s, the childhood obesity rate was four to six percent. This dramatic increase is a result of more junk food, bigger portions and less physical activity. All of this leads to an increase in high blood pressure, asthma, Type 2 diabetes and an increase in adult obesity. These are crazy things to be worried about for kids. In addition, there is a lack of effort put forth by schools for physical activities and lunch-room menus. Things need to change or, for the first time in two centuries, life expectancy is going to start shortening.

Where to find more Information:

- *Health Consequences of Childhood Obesity - http://womenshealth.aetna.com*
- *Childhood Obesity: Make weight loss a family affair - www.mayoclinic.com*
- *Report: Obesity will reverse life expectancy gains - www.cnn.com*
- *www.obesity.org*

FIT TIP #95

Joy From Soy?

A few years ago, soy became a staple in many diets because studies showed that it lowered bad cholesterol, raised good cholesterol, protected your bones and lowered the risk of cancer. Lately, studies have shown that they may have overestimated these claims. But wait before you run to throw the tofu out! Just because it isn't capable of doing all those things doesn't mean that it can't be beneficial to your diet. Using soy as a substitute for less healthy foods as well as enjoying soy burgers, edamame and soy milk are all good things. Even though soy isn't the miracle we hoped for, you can still receive some of the benefits that were previously claimed.

Where to find more Information:

- *The Benefits of Soy - http://health.discovery.com*
- *The Healing Power of Soy's Isoflavones - www.fwhc.org*

Blood Sugar

When people talk about eliminating sugary snacks and watching their blood sugar, it isn't just to prevent excess weight. A diet high in sugar can cause problems for more than just your waistline down the road. It can lead to heart disease, stroke and diabetes. To help yourself in this fight, try to resist the urge to hit the simple sugar snacks for an energy boost. Things like candy bars, cupcakes and fancy coffee drinks will all give you an energy spike, but then will allow you to crash. This will just leave you wanting more sugar.

Where to find more Information:

- *Women's Health Magazine, April 2007*

FIT TIP #97

Watermelon Temperature

One of the best summer treats is watermelon. Here is a tip for you to take advantage of all the lycopene that watermelon offers. When you buy a whole, uncut watermelon keep it at room temperature until you are ready to eat it. Then chill it in the fridge before cutting, so you can enjoy it nice and cool. After cutting it, you need to put it in the fridge. Keeping it at room temperature, up until cutting it, will keep all its nutrients at full strength.

Where to find more Information:

- *The Best Watermelon May Not Be The Coldest - http://query.nytimes.com*

Alcohol Tolerance

Is there such a thing as an alcohol tolerance level? The more you drink alcohol, the more you need to drink to feel the same effects. This is known as your alcohol tolerance. BUT, your blood alcohol concentration does not vary as your tolerance increases. This means that one drink will always be the same in your bloodstream. This tolerance makes it harder for those who drink regularly to accurately monitor their impairment. What use to take three beers to feel the effects, now takes five. The same is not true of your motor skills and this includes driving. The body normally processes one drink per hour, so any more than that, despite how you feel will be considered driving under the influence.

FIT TIP #99

Where to find more Information:

- *Alcohol Tolerance Associated with Family History - www.sciencedaily.com*
- *Alcohol and Tolerance - www.about.com*

Brand vs. Generic

What is the difference between brand name and generic prescription drugs? After my research, it looks like the cost really is the big difference. The FDA has to approve generics just as they do brand names. The generics have to be chemically equivalent and therapeutically equivalent, so it doesn't seem like there is much room for error. However, I have read that the absorption rate could differ in hormonal drugs, like thyroid, birth control, and others. Many times doctors will prescribe the brand name for a reason on these medications. If the doctor specifies a brand name, a pharmacist has to fill it with the brand name unless they consult with the doctor. Brand names are so expensive because the original company has to do all the initial research, advertising and testing. After their seven year patent runs out, the recipe is up for grabs.

Where to find more Information:

- *Generic Drugs: Saving Money at the Pharmacy - www.ftc.gov*
- *How to Know Which Direction to Take - www.rxdirect.com*
- *Cracking the Code - www.oag.state.md.us*

The Standard

It's too cold, it's raining, I didn't sleep well, I'm hungry, I forgot my iPod, the gym will be crowded, I'm on the other side of town.... and on and on. If you find yourself saying these things to prevent a workout then you are normal. For some reason, we put working out on a pedestal and require only the best of circumstances in order to follow through and actually workout. This might be because we are always looking for an excuse to skip out. If you use an excuse enough, it starts to have validity and then every time it looks like rain it will mean that you can't workout. To change this habit means you have to change the standard so that there is no excuse to skip a workout. If it's cold- layer up, if you are tired- it will boost your energy. If you try hard enough, you will find that there is always an excuse to workout so reverse your thinking and get moving.

Notes

Use the following section to keep notes of things you would like to accomplish, tips you found interesting or comments you would like to send back to Amy Mac at www.withamymac.com.

_____

_____

_____

_____

_____

_____

_____

_____

_____

_____

_____

_____

_____

"The secret of getting ahead is getting started. The secret of getting started is breaking your complex overwhelming tasks into small manageable tasks, and then starting on the first one." *- Mark Twain*

About Amy Mac

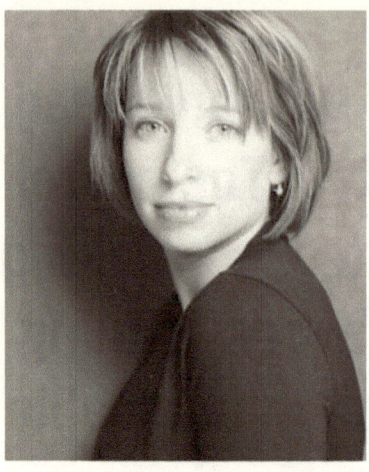

I am a certified personal trainer from San Diego State, NASM, Scirion Institute, APEX and AFAA for group exercise. I also have a BS in Organizational Leadership and Supervision from Purdue University. I've been a hip hop and jazz dancer and choreographer, I've taught dance classes, been a coxswain for Purdue Crew and was a nationally competing cheerleader in school. I've always been active and attribute that to my attraction to fitness.

My Podcasts

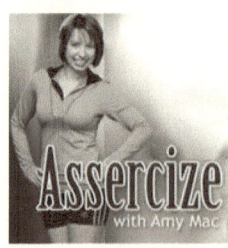

Assercize

This show is a spin-off from a segment on Adam Curry's Daily Source Code podcast. Each week you will be coached through a different butt-sculpting exercise by Certified Personal Trainer, Amy Mac. Dedicated to giving you that perfect booty you have always wanted, this show is quick and to the point. Listen to this 3 minute audio show at home, at work or at the gym and learn new and different ways to sculpt your buns.

Website: *http://assercize.podshow.com*
Subscribe: *http://feeds.feedburner.com/assercize*

My Podcasts

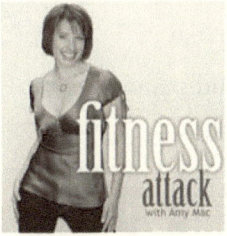

Fitness Attack

This podcast is your gateway to becoming healthy and staying fit. Served up in 60 second doses, I bring years of knowledge and experience to this short format show. I do extensive research, providing links to relevant sources in order to bring the most up to date information. Leaving no topic behind, I cover everything from dieting tips, little known health facts about previously discouraged food items, product reviews, honest reviews of food, technology, personal health, urban fitness myths and much more. User questions are always accepted and researched for future episodes. All tips from this book have come from this podcast.

> **Website**: *http://fitness.podshow.com*
> **Subscribe**: *http://feeds.feedburner.com/wam*

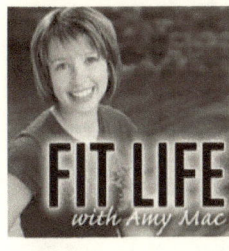

Fit Life

If you have ever said, "There has got to be a better way to do this," then this show is for you. I have that same thought everyday and so I decided to create a show for that purpose. This show is focused around YOU living a fit life. I talk about news & trends, do a gear review, demonstrate an exercise, delve into foods and recipes and of course, I give you a health and fitness tip. I want this to be your all inclusive guide to making you AND your life better. This means suggestions are welcome. If you have ever wanted to see an exercise demonstrated, wondered how to eat that strange vegetable in the produce aisle or curious about gear, gadgets and fitness equipment, now is your chance to have me find the answer.

> **Website**: *http://fitlife.podshow.com*
> **Subscribe**: *http://feeds.feedburner.com/fitlife*

More Information

For more information on any of these topics, you can visit the resources listed below each tip. You can also visit *www.WithAmyMac.com* to subscribe to my audio and video shows, as well as news, recipe cards and other downloads, so you can get your daily dose of health and fitness info.

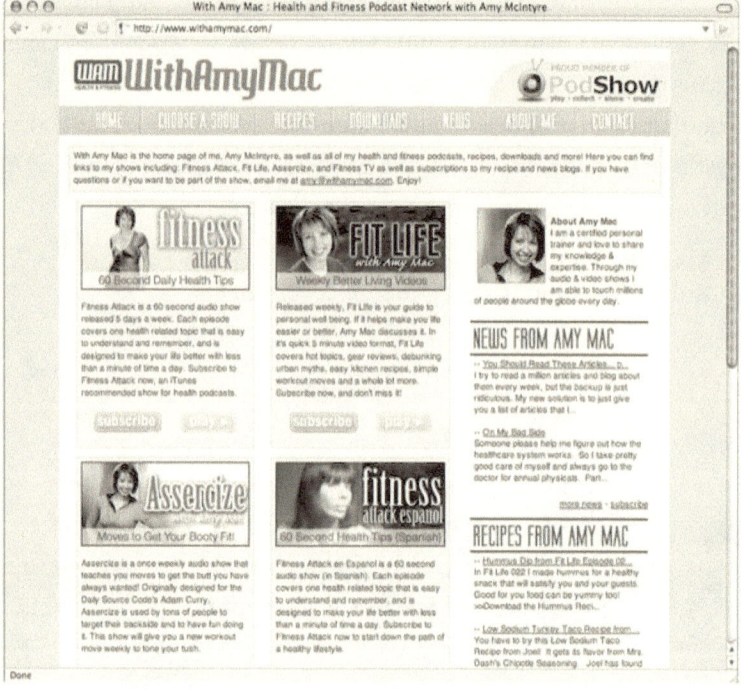

All of my shows are hosted on the PodShow Network. They have generously provided hosting, support, promotion and advertising. You can support my show by supporting PodShow. Create your own account at *www.PodShow.com* and find other great shows, just like mine.

www.ingramcontent.com/pod-product-compliance
Lightning Source LLC
Chambersburg PA
CBHW020301290526
45784CB00003B/1326